NATURE LIVING TOWARDS A BETTER HEALTH.

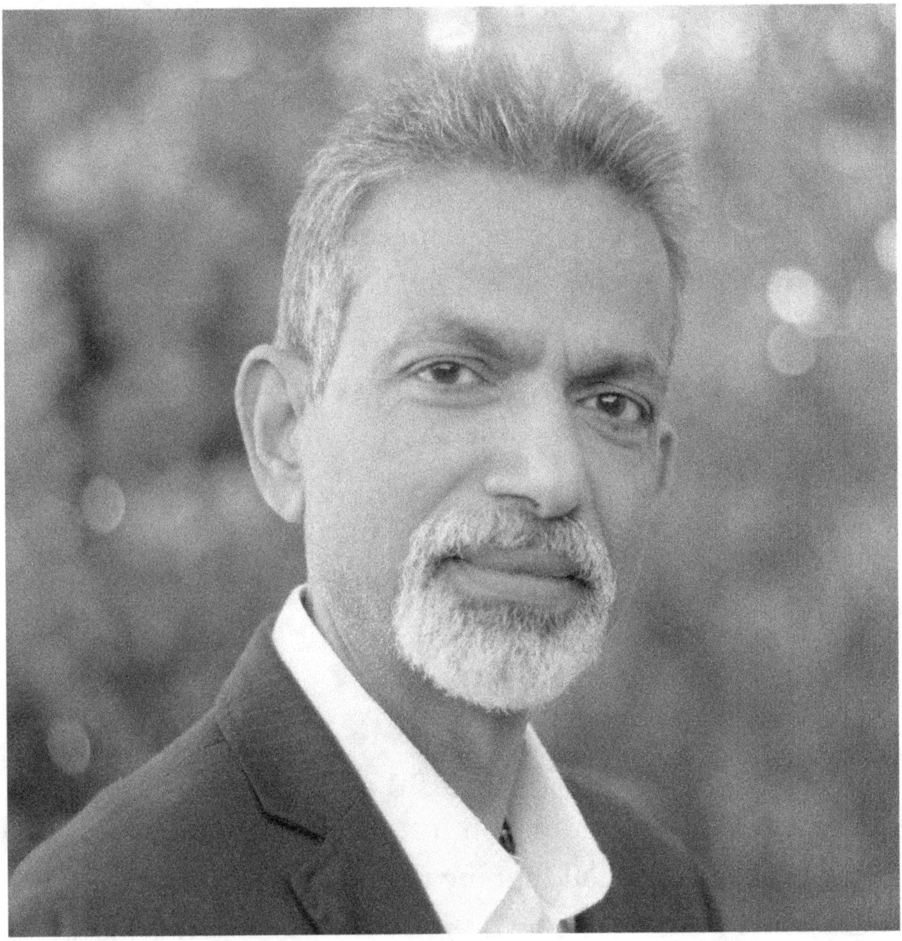

George Varughese

Live a life Medicine Free, Disease free, the Nature way with your own Vital Power. Find your own Vital power, freedom and tranquility. This book will guide you in your life journey to reach the shore of peace and will help you to define your own story if you are ready.

Preface

My long search and journey for a reliable healing therapy helped me to reach to Natural healing ideas which I want to share for a greater benefit for those searching for a healthy life practice. My search was to find solution for my problems but I am sure while sharing my experience that will help the enthusiast to find a better path to cure many diseases in our life journey. We witness tall claims from many therapies and practices around us but until we get involved, experienced and analysis we won't get the right weight of each therapy.

When I was young and healthy my requirement was quick fix for any pain, flu or discomfort as quickly as possible. I found and experienced that those quick fixing was the beginning or pathway for future health issues. We should be wise and in control over our nature powered ever building, growing and transforming human body. I would advise that it is not wise to go for any quick fix for any of our health related issues because our body is a self-growing self-repairing phenomena which is self-grown and formed organism developed from a single cell.

My experience could benefit many and especially the youngsters and enthusiastic to attain a better health rather than be cheated with many false ideas prevailing in our modern fast paced society. We have only one life and if we lose the health we will end up in a care place living with someone's mercy. We should have a control over our own health and life rather than future dependency on medicine, machine or a third person.

The system of Nature healing is an ancient Vedic knowledge used by many in India for centuries and lives a healthy life. Natural way of life has been practiced by Indians for many centuries but it is only followed by few people who eagerly or wisely seeks it. Nature way of life demands a lot a self-discipline and well control over our temptations over food, drinks and habits.

The inspiration to write this book is dedicated to some social activists from USA, whom I met on their visit to India in January 2014. They were eagerly seeking to learn about this therapy but they could not get a comprehensive idea about this treatment and the opportunities of it because of the language barrier and their short stay in those places.

While reading this book you will find that there is a way towards a healthy life without the intervention of any chemical medications. Those who want a muscular body and those involving sports may not be able to accept these ideas until they fall sick. The nature way of life is for those who love an ordinary life style according to the rhythm of our environment and those who eagerly seeking happiness and tranquility. If you want a diseases free life for you and your children or dear ones it is a good book to get a new direction and hope.

The idea of this book which is the result of my life journey with encounters of disease and the experience of experiments and challenges. Many portions are being translated from various Naturopathy books, sources and it is mentioned in the main frame accordingly and in bibliography.

My Story

I do not know where to start my story of my pilgrimage to find a solution to the health issues which is an inevitable part in our life journey. My first doctor was my friend. When I had a simple headache he advised me to have a pain killer; it helped and the pain is relived. Then it was my solution; whenever there is a headache the pain killers were my fortress, it was easily available in many stores and reachable without any prescription or advice. The frequency of the use of pain killers has increased and its side effects has not bothered me since my body is healthy enough to withstand its poisoning.

After few years of the hectic life I was diagnosed with high blood pressure at a young age of 36. Then the GP prescribed me to start a tablet or drug for higher BP, by then I am under two medications; regular BP medicine and occasional pain killers. With these two medicines I knew it is being restricted not cured. As long as it is being restricted I am capable to perform my occupation, I was not much concerned and did not search for a lasting solution. After 8 years of regular anti-hypertensive and occasional painkillers, medical test revealed that my Kidney functions are not normal and I was facing a problem. Doctor advised me to take care but they did not have any therapy to improve the kidney function nor had any medicine to control the diseases progression. Lab test after two years shows that my liver function also being elevated with GGT and ALP but again there is no medication in Allopathy to restrict the progression.

Few years passed, time was running, my diseases progressed and still no cure to my problems. I have searched for other famous therapies like Ayurveda and Chinese medicines. Both these people have treated me with their therapies but my problem was still steadily increasing and getting worse. For two years I have taken Ayurveda medicines for lever functions and Chinese acupuncture done for one month for Kidney improvement; but still I did not have a cure. I have consulted with some of my Indian friends and they have advised some dried leaves infusion which could improve the that helped me. Finally, a cousin of mine advise me to try the Nature life therapy. I have researched and found that many people are cured for various diseases and thought this may help me.

Nature life hospital was a new experience for me, it transformed me to think and to revise my past experience. It helped me to think and rewind what I should have done for a healthy life. I want to share this experience with my fellow being for your health as well as your children's. Your health is your business do not give control of your health to anyone else. I have not found any big reception and welcoming people in Nature life hospital, like many five-star Allopathy hospitals elsewhere, they were just ordinary people helping you to heal if you are willing to co-operate.

They went through my medical report and told me my disease is not completely curable but it can be controlled with strict diet. For my vitamin D deficiency, they advised me to have morning and evening sunshine and there is no need to consume any vitamin D tablets. They asked me to stop the Resonium A allopathy medicine to control high potassium in my blood reading and gave me some vegetable juice to drink. I was concerned that my Potassium may increase without a medicine but later on I found they were right because they had the experience and past data to be sure and off course it proved to be right for me.

After reaching the Naturopathy wellness center on the 4th day of my stay I had to stop the anti-hypertensive drug I was taking for almost 18 years. Last two years I am living without any kind of medication and that amazing story I want to share with my readers. In the following chapters I would like to bring some of the truth in the Nature way of life. Some in India say that this as Gandhian way of life because it was followed by Gandhi during his life time. Also it is the ancient Vedic way of life followed by many and it is not very popular because of its strict dietary requirements.

Hard lessons I have learned

This book will help you to analysis and choose the best when you have illness. Or you can choose the best for a better life from the hard lessons I have learned. Life is short and we can't gamble or ignore it we should be able to pick the best. It is a question mark who will guide us towards a better life? I have tried all the available therapies around the world and found the best way to prevent many of the illness is Nature way of life.

None of the therapy system can claim to cure all the disease, some are good in few and others can do better in other diseases. Unfortunately, Allopathy is not recognizing the relevance of other existing therapies for various reasons. Ayurveda, Chines herbal medicines and Homeopathic are relevant in some cases but they are not even claiming to cure all disease. Then a natural question will arise where to approach for the best practice?

I found the answer from Nature healing system; turn back to your own Vital Power of your body and help heal many of your disease naturally by your own Vital Power, yourself. It can be attained through self -discipline and food control. Food is the best medicine for healing, food can kill and food can heal all depends on how wisely you use it. Most of the discussion and ideas are simple but only for those who can discipline their mind and temptation towards food can attain the best from Nature way of life.

How to approach Sickness

While reading the whole book you will be able to understand what are the main sickness which affects our body and how it is being developed and how to approach them wisely to cure it. The medication will be minimal and you will be able to choose the food, medicine and therapy according your diseases and requirements.

In this modern age we are spending most of our saving in a life time to treat our sickness during the ageing process or treat our children when they are young. Our general understanding is that all sicknesses are destructive which will destroy our life. Once we are sick we will approach the immediate available therapy to destroy the sickness with the help of medicine and that is the common man's approach; most of the cases the patient will be cured and some cases that could be the end of the life for that person.

Now we have many Allopathic hospitals in most of the cities and urban areas. There are other therapies like Ayurveda, Chinese Herbal & Acupuncture, Homeopathy, Unani and local traditional way of healing through other herbal treatments which are still prevalent in many remote communities around the Globe. All these therapies have proven to be effective for many diseases and none of these are good for every sickness. Now we have reached an age with much medical and scientific equipment for diagnose and therapeutic purposes. We are capable of assessing most of the sickness and treat in time. But again in some countries because of the government funding and private medical cover; we found a new trend that is over treating a sick patient in many cases.

Keeping all these in mind let us approach our sickness and therapy in an ancient way which is the nature way of healing. Here we will find a way of Natural healing with our vital power. Also we have to examine whether medicine can play any major role in the healing process for many of our problems or our Vital Power can heal the sickness.

Classification of sickness by Naturopathy

Acute, Chronic & Degenerative disease are the main three classification of sickness defined by some of the Naturopathy Gurus. In Naturopathy the Acute has been classified as the sickness which is very visible but less harmful like Flu, Fever, Headache, Stomach pain vomiting etc. Whereas Migraine, Asthma, BP, Rheumatic fever, Diabetics, Psoriasis, Ulcer these kind of diseases are Chronic disease. The degenerative diseases are Cancer, AIDS, Kidney disease, Lever problems, TB etc and advanced heart disease can also be included in the third category.

Why naturopathy is classifying these diseases into these categories? The treatment approach for each category should be different. Every disease can't be treated in the same manner. Ultimately while our body is encountering these diseases, it will resist or repair as it can at various stages. Naturopathy helps through various measures to empower the body to repair or resist these diseases using its vital power. *[Dr. N Venkitakrishnanpotty, book- Achieve Complete Health Through Disease]*

What Naturopathy can do

I would briefly discuss what are the challenges to the growth of Naturopathy therapy first. Many alternative therapies to Allopathy exists in various cultures but those therapies are not being widely published or caught the attention for various reasons. Clinically successful or acceptance with the recipients are not being brought to the lime light because many of the therapies do not have the backing of private medical insurance companies or government medical boards. Most of the medical boards are being governed by Allopathy practitioners so support for alternative medicine will be minimal or nil.

Now there is a question arise naturally, are these treatments for the patients wellbeing or for the pleasure of few people who run the therapy industry? Who will stand up for the rights of common man to choose the right therapies for the patients or the beneficiaries of these services? Who will voice out for the rights of the tax payers for a best cure for their diseases? Now it is the high time to think for the right therapies for the illness, especially if one system cannot heal an illness there should be a way out for other available therapies anywhere in the world which is effective for those illness. Let us look what Naturopathy or herbal medicine in some countries can do where other system can't help healing.

How does Naturopathy Work?

Naturopathy encourages patients to become active participants in the therapy through understanding of the strengths and weaknesses of their own body and taking responsibility for their own actions. This system will teach the participant how to attain their wellbeing through adopting beneficial lifestyle habits. The most important thing is educating the participant and an individualized eating plans, and regularly participating in activities which aid relaxation for a mind and body's participation in stress reduction and self-care. Naturopathy teaches that the human body is constituted with five elements; Earth, Water, Sunlight, Air and Ether [Aakash]; it is a complex representation of all immediate forces of nature surrounding to us.

Naturopathy is not an alternative medicine-prescribed therapy. There were few people from the west has advocated for Naturopathy in the past. Sir Isaac Jennings asked a question many decades ago why a sick person should be poisoned more than should a well person; and I do not believe the world will endure until he finds such a reason. He advocated that there are but two medical systems in existence--the Drug Medical System and the Hygienic Medical System. Other prominent advocates in the past were Herbert Shelton, John H Tildone, R T Thrall and so on. Meantime India had many Naturopathy Gurus in the beginning of the 20th Century like Mahatma Gandhi,

Acharya Laxman and later on their disciples in many parts of the country to enhance and propagate this system.

There are many Naturopathy practices existing but not widely practiced or popularized. Indian Naturopathy and Chinese naturopathies are some of the main stream but herbal medicines like Ayurveda and other local knowledge are still prevalent in many societies. We know we had a very effective herbal medicine treatment available in villages of Kerala State in India for Hepatitis **B** but unfortunately these knowledge is not being properly being taught or preserved for future generations. They have not sold or propagated their knowledge for monetary benefits or for their personal esteem.

What Indian Naturopathy Teaches?

Sri RR Varma the famous Indian Naturopathy doctor says in his book why nature cure is a triumph when other therapies fail with some diseases. Nature cure facilitates to utilize the vital power of our own body. Naturopathy can cure many diseases like simple flu, fever, diabetics, Psoriasis and heart block where other therapies fails.

All the living being has the vital power to grow, sustain and diminish after a certain time and that is the nature's power of creation of the organism. We can find this nature's power in a small seed which is sprouting and growing into a big tree, sustains and reproduces fruits and nuts. This is what happens in all living beings in our surrounding and it is a continues process due to natures vital power.

When a human egg splits--first into 2, then 4, then 8, 16, 32, 64, and so on--it embarks on a venture that will, over the next nine months, produce descendant cells with a huge variety of shapes and functions: bone cells, nerve cells, red and white blood cells; the cells of the eyes, fingernails, stomach, and skin. Once a human body develops it has the vital power for reproduction also and it is a continues process like a chain. Vital power of our body will build the body for 25 year sustain it for another 25 years and will help to diminish or destroy for the next 25 years, which is the nature's rule.
[Ref, Sri. R R Varma, book, Sugham Sathyam, Rogam Midhya]

Remedy for a simple flu and cough.

Here I would like to bring some of the understanding of a Nature cure doctor for the benefit of our readers. Also let us check how Allopathy approach and treat this illness. Also let us look at this illness with details and how these therapies are treating this illness.

Reasons and approaches of Nature cure treatment for Flu

Common flu is an occasional visitor in our life for majority of the population but many of us are not taking this flue very seriously. There is a common saying that if we take medicine that will cured in one week if no medicine it will be cured in 7 days. In allopathy there is no proper medicine for this simple disease. The main cause of the flu is many known and unknown virus and that is the finding of science.

Naturopathy approaches this problem in a very different way. How does this flu develop in our body? How do this cough and mucus develop in our body? Naturopathy treatment tries to eradicate or stop the root cause of the problem not merely treating the visible sign of the problem.

Naturopathy and Ayurveda have almost the same view on flu and its treatment. Cooked food, wrong combination of food intake, excessive quantity of food, wrong eating time, late night food intake etc. are the main cause of flu. When body wants to clear the mucus and cleanse the body which is stored in various parts of the body it is finding a way out through the flu process; it is not a disease but it is a uncomfortable process for the body to keep it clean and healthy. If we are ready to co-operate with our body's Vital Power in this cleaning process it will get over very fast.

The best way is to abstain from our daily work and take complete rest; rest means no TV, no reading just bed rest and your vital power will use the whole energy to restore your health. This will help you to repair and restore your energy and you will be back to action very soon. Whereas Allopathy interrupt that process with medicine; once you are consuming medicine in a sick state it is a double work for our system to cleanse the chemical supplied in the form of medicine and it will be a prolonged and difficult task for our vital power to cleanse and repair any damaged cells or parts.

Flu information

A productive cough produces phlegm or mucus (sputum). The mucus may have drained down the back of the throat from the nose or sinuses or may have come up from the lungs. A productive cough generally should not be suppressed-it clears mucus from the lungs. There are many causes of a productive cough, such as:

- Viral illnesses. It is normal to have a productive cough when you have a <u>common cold</u>. Coughing is often triggered by mucus that drains down the back of the throat.
- Infections. An infection of the lungs or upper airway passages can cause a cough. A productive cough may be a symptom of <u>pneumonia</u>, <u>bronchitis</u>, <u>sinusitis</u>, or <u>tuberculosis</u>.
- Chronic <u>lung disease</u>. A productive cough could be a sign that a disease such as <u>chronic obstructive pulmonary disease</u> (<u>COPD</u>) is getting worse or that you have an infection.
- <u>Stomach</u> acid backing up into the <u>esophagus</u> . This type of coughing may be a symptom of <u>gastroesophageal reflux disease</u> (<u>GERD</u>) and may awaken you from <u>sleep</u>.

- Nasal discharge (underline postnasal drip) draining down the back of the throat. This can cause a productive cough or the feeling that you constantly need to clear your throat. Experts disagree about whether a postnasal drip or the viral illness that caused it is responsible for the cough.
- Smoking or other tobacco use. Productive coughs in a person who smokes or uses other forms of tobacco is often a sign of lung damage or irritation of the throat or esophagus

[http://www.webmd.com/cold-and-flu/tc/coughs-topic-overview]

Flu Problem facing in USA alone.

Each year, approximately 5 to 20 percent of Americans come down with the flu. Although most recover without incident, flu-related complications result in more than 200,000 hospitalizations and between 3,000 and 49,000 deaths each year. Colds generally do not cause serious complications, but they are among the leading reasons for visiting a doctor and for missing school or work.

Some people try natural products such as herbs or vitamins and minerals to prevent or treat these illnesses. But do they really work? What does the science say?

[https://nccih.nih.gov/health/tips/flucold.htm]

Official NHS advice which advises flu sufferers to take paracetamol has been contradicted by a new medical study.

The popular drug – which is a key ingredient in many cold and flu remedies – had no success reducing fever or other symptoms like aches and pains, academics found.

Analysis of the results, published in the journal *Respirology*, said there was no significant difference in body temperature between 40 flu sufferers given paracetamol for five days and 40 who were given placebos.

In this study, paracetamol was not harmful, but we also found that paracetamol was not beneficial either."
Dr Irene Braithwaite

[http://www.telegraph.co.uk/news/science/12048064/Paracetamol-for-the-flu-has-no-effect-say-scientists.html]

Remedy for headache

Headache can occur for various reasons; bloating, undigested food, excessive day light exposure and heat, high or low BP, mental strains etc. are some of the reasons for simple headache. Generally, these simple headaches are the problems related to other parts of the body not head. Tea, coffee or any kind of pain killers are the immediate quick fix for these problem, which many follow but this is an unhealthy practice. Headache is a signal by the brain to indicate any other problem existing in our body, if we can find a solution to that problem then the headache will disappear.

The best remedy for headache is to cooldown your head with a wet towel or cold water but not ice cold. Also take a wet cloth to bind around your stomach. If the headache is due to bloating or heaviness in stomach, then take an enema with clean lukewarm water and clean up your colon and bowel. Bowel enemas are a natural therapy modality followed by Mahatma Gandhi and his disciples and he used to promote that for a balanced mind and health. Until the headache is clear do not eat any cooked food, fresh fruit juice is the best option.

Remedy for a fever

Do not be panic when you get a fever. This is body's cleansing process of our Vital power to remove the contaminations which we have received through our food, water or from our environment. The Vital power increases the temperature with great difficulty to repair our problems so do not attempt to reduce the temperature if it is only 102 degrees. If the temperature is climbing above 102 then tie a wet cloth on head and around stomach. Do not do any kind of work in this difficult time of the body and let us co-operate with our Vital power to repair it with proper rest.

Also it is very important to fast and keep away from all other physical activities including reading and watching TV. You can only have some fruit juice that preferably fresh orange juice will be the best. Here it is very important to note the words of Hippoceates that give me a power to produce fever I will cure all diseases, he is trying to say that fever is just a natural process of cleansing the body it is not a disease it is a blessing if we approach that wisely. Meantime the yellow fever and rheumatic fever are not under this category. [ref book, Nature Life Thoughts, Sri. R R Varma]

Cure for Hypertension or BP

Causes of Hypertension

Major causes of hypertension are modern fast paced lifestyle and stress. If stress continues for a long periods of time, pressure may get permanently raised. Excessive intake of intoxicants, smoking, excessive consumption of tea &coffee, processed foods etc. could cause BP. Obesity, hardening of arteries, severe constipation and diabetes also lead to high blood pressure. Consuming excessive painkillers, common salt, Fat-rich food items also cause blood pressure to increase. [http://naturopathycure.com/Naturopathy-for-High-Blood-Pressure-or-Hypertension.php]

Naturopathy have a great healing approach towards BP. Hypertension can be controlled if we are ready to control our diets. Lifestyle plays an important role in treating high blood pressure. If you are successful in taking control of your blood pressure with a healthy lifestyle you will avoid the medication which can save your Liver, Kidney and Heart and will be able to avoid many other future concerns.

Diet is the most important thing we should follow to bring the blood pressure under control. Check how many times you are consuming food or drink in a day. Yoga gurus say that two times of food in a day is often good for men. Naturopathy gurus say two times cooked food and one time fruits is an ideal diet for human being.

When you select fruit, avoid mixing acid fruits with sweet fruits as this may create problems for the digestion process. Cooked food means vegetarian food is always good for people with BP, occasional non-vegetarian may not be harmful if you are young but when you are getting old or already crossed 50 years of age reduce the intake of non-vegetarian and high protein diet if you have still high BP. Raw vegetables are recommended for hypertension patients. Cabbage, Spinach, Tomatoes, Cucumber, Onion, Radish should be consumed raw; lemon juice and little salt could be added for taste. *[Ref, Sri. R R Varma, book, Sugham Sathyam, Rogam Midhya]*

Regular yoga or light exercise can lower the blood pressure; walking, jogging, cycling, swimming or dancing could be selected according to your life style. If the diet and exercise are in control your emotions and stress will be under control, then you can easily manage your BP.

Naturopathy Successfully Treats Heart block, Diabetes, Psoriasis & Epilepsy

The treatment for Heart block, Diabetics, Psoriasis and Epilepsy are very successful with Indian Naturopathy. But we cannot explain all those treatments here for few reasons. Firstly, each of these problems should be treated for quite sometimes and the patient should be under supervision and care with trained and responsible Naturopathy health professionals. There are no home solutions for these problems but once you are treated you will learn a new life and how to live a Nature way of life.

With experience we know that there is no Allopathy medicine developed to cure any of these above diseases still they will treat the patients. After a prolong treatment under Allopathy medicine all these above categories of diseases will be worsened for most of the patients. We know that many of the diabetic's patients have lost their leg towards their older age or some stage that is the Allopathy treatment whereas Naturopathy can cure diabetics. Heart blocks, Psoriasis, and Epilepsy patients are getting a complete cure and a new life through Naturopathy treatments.

A strict diet will slowly help our Vital Power and our body's Vital Power is the doctor/healer. Under supervision in a Naturopathy hospital in India one can get a complete cure for all the above diseases but we have to sacrifice our fast pace life for a Nature way of life and should be able to follow the diet according to the program advice.

Traditional Chinese Medicine & Acupuncture.

Chinese herbal medicine is an essential part of the healing system and is known as Traditional Chinese Medicine (TCM). TMC includes acupuncture, massage dietary advice and exercise. It is a popular method of treatment throughout the world these days, with nearly three million Australians visiting TCM practitioners every year.

The basic principles of this therapy is very different from traditional Western notions about health, illness and the workings of the body. Chinese herbs are prescribed to normalize imbalanced energy of the body, or Qi (pronounced 'chee'), that runs through invisible meridians in the body. Studies have shown Chinese herbal medicines to be successful in treating a range of disorders, particularly gynecological and gastrointestinal disorders

Things to Remember when using Chinese Herbs

- Chinese herbal medicine is the essential part of a larger healing system called Traditional Chinese Medicine.
- Herbs are prescribed to restore energy balance to the opposing forces of energy - Yin and Yang - that run through invisible channels in the body.
- Herbs can act on the body as powerfully as pharmaceutical drugs and should be treated with the same caution and respect of Allopathy.

[https://www.betterhealth.vic.gov.au/health/conditionsandtreatments/chinese-herbal-medicine]

US National institute of Mental Health is funding research into use of Acupuncture for Bipolar Disorder to be carried out at UT South-western Medical Centre at Dallas. The study that involves 30 patients aims whether the acupuncture can reduce the medication of these patients.

The U K's metal health foundation has proposed acupuncture should be made more available to depressed patients. They carried out an investigation of ear acupuncture and its potential benefits for woman with mental health problems. Most of them are benefited and two women came off anti-depressant after getting this treatment.

What WHO found on Acupuncture

In an official report, *Acupuncture: Review and Analysis of Reports on Controlled Clinical Trials*, the WHO (WHO) has listed the following symptoms, diseases and conditions that have been shown through controlled trials to be treated effectively by acupuncture:

- low back pain
- neck pain
- sciatica
- tennis elbow
- knee pain
- periarthritis of the shoulder
- sprains
- facial pain (including craniomandibular disorders)
- headache
- dental pain
- tempromandibular (TMJ) dysfunction
- rheumatoid arthritis
- induction of labor
- correction of malposition of fetus (breech presentation)
- morning sickness
- nausea and vomiting
- postoperative pain
- stroke
- essential hypertension
- primary hypotension
- renal colic
- leucopenia
- adverse reactions to radiation or chemotherapy
- allergic rhinitis, including hay fever
- biliary colic
- depression (including depressive neurosis and depression following stroke)

- acute bacillary dysentery
- primary dysmenorrhea
- acute epigastralgia
- peptic ulcer

[http://www.acupuncturetoday.com/archives2004/oct/10amaro.html]

Ayurveda the Indian Science

Indian Ayurveda is an ancient Vedic system of Therapy. The word "Ayurveda" is translated from Sanskrit means the science of life. Ayurveda is a non-symptomatic medicine says Peter Gowan from the Australasian Ayurvedic Practitioners Association. Meditation is just one of the most powerful tools the ancient Ayurvedic physicians prescribed for balancing the mind and body - See more at:

http://www.chopra.com/ccl/what-is-ayurveda#sthash.HVHbU7jj.dpuf

Defining that human beings are part of nature, Ayurveda describes three basic energies that govern our inner and outer environments: movement, transformation, and structure. Known in Sanskrit as Vata (Wind), Pitta (Fire), and Kapha (Earth), these primary forces are responsible for the characteristics of our mind and body. Each of us has a unique proportion of these three forces that shapes our nature. If Vata is dominant in our system, we tend to be thin, light, enthusiastic, energetic, and changeable.

Ayurveda & Hepatitis B

Hepatitis B is growing as a challenge to many communities around the world and Ayurveda has found a break through recently and it could be useful for those who are interested and not egoistic. [This information derived from their website]

Clinical and laboratory research from India has proven that an Ayurvedic formula used for liver infections halts the often deadly hepatitis B virus. The researchers utilized a formula that has been referred to as HD-03/ES. This is an Ayurvedic herb liver formulation made up of the extracts of two herbs: Cyperus rotundus (also referred to as Java grass or Nut grass) and Cyperus scariosus (referred to as Cypriol or Nagarmotha).

The researchers tested four different concentrations of this herbal combination against the hepatitis B surface antigens using liver cells (PLC/PRF/5) infected with hepatitis and actually carcinogenic.

The cultures were tested for 24 hours each and then underwent enzyme assays to determine the results. In all four concentrations, which ranged from 125 micrograms per milliliter to 1000 micrograms – the herbal extract suppressed the cells' ability to produce the hepatitis B surface antigens – which allow the virus to infect other cells.

http://www.realnatural.org/ayurvedic-herbal-formula-proven-to-halt-hepatitis-b-virus/

The research also found that that combination downgraded the ability of the HBV-infected cells' DNA to replicate. This of course is necessary for the virus to stay alive.

Evolution of Allopathy treatment.

Louis Pasteur founder of germ theory has developed vaccinations for diseases such as anthrax, cholera, TB and smallpox. The scientific communities researched in line with louis Pasteur's Germ theory to find solution for all the illness we encounter and later on found bacteria is the cause of some of the illness. Still Allopathy do not have a remedy to many illnesses like basic flue, heart disease, cancer, kidney imparities etc.

Medical Scientist are still in good progress to achieve the best result for therapies for many challenges we face. Many people die in their young age due to illness which can't be treated effectively in time. There are no proper answers to Heart disease and Diabetic in Allopathy; still they continue to treat these patients. In both these cases Allopathy has a mechanical cutting and fixing approach towards an ever rebuilding and reshaping Human body. We found none of the prescribed medicine can improve the condition of a diabetic patient rather it worsens after a prolong Allopathic medicine. Also Psoriasis condition can't be treated or cured by Allopathy.

India Banned some of the popular drugs as following.

Indian Government has banned the popular medicine which sold in India for decades for flu, fever and headache Vicks Action 500. FMCG firm Procter and Gamble (P&G) has discontinued manufacture and sale of its popular brand 'Vicks Action 500 Extra' with immediate effect after the government banned fixed dose combination drugs. The list of banned items in this week alone is more than 300 and still 500 more drugs are in scrutiny.

"The Government of India has prohibited the manufacture for sale, sale and distribution of fixed dose combination drugs (Paracetamol + Phenylephrine + Caffeine) with immediate effect," Pfizer said in a BSE filing.

It further said: "Our product 'Vicks Action 500 Extra' has the same fixed dose combination and gets covered under notification. we have discontinued the manufacture and sale of all SKUs of 'Vicks Action 500 Extra with immediate effect." Yesterday, drug majors Pfizer and Abbott stopped sale of their popular cough syrups Corex and Phensedyl respectively, after the government banned over 300 fixed dose combinations (FDCs) drugs.

[http://www.moneycontrol.com/news/business/pg-stops-salevicks-action-500-extra-after-govt-ban_5877321.html]

http://www.cdsco.nic.in/forms/list.aspx?lid=2028&Id=31

Conclusion

Indian Naturopathy is a Vedic knowledge and practitioners are taking this as a service to the community. It is so ancient and the knowledge was so wide spread until the beginning of 20th century. The arrival of Allopathy and its quick reliefs has created less acceptance to the common man who want a quick fix. But these days the intellectuals and the modern man has taken a great interest to rediscover the true value of that ancient Vedic knowledge. It's a harmless or non-violent approach towards our own system and empowering our Vital power would be a truly acceptable practice.

Naturopathy is teaching us or creating a life style; educating the participant with an individualized eating plans, and regularly participating in activities which aid relaxation for a mind and body's participation in stress reduction and self-care. Naturopathy has a holistic approach to human body which constitutes of five elements; Earth, Water, Sunlight, Air and Ether/Akash. These five elements are a complex representation of all immediate forces of nature, surrounding us and makes an essential contact with us on a daily basis.

Naturopathy is becoming increasingly popular in all countries across the globe, especially among those who want to escape the various side effects and symptoms caused by the allopathic system of medicine. Many passages are taken from many Naturopathy books written in Malayalam language and it is mostly the translation for the benefit of the readers and the name of the book and authors names are mentioned on those areas. There are many other ailments that can be cured by Naturopathy treatment, which I have not mentioned here and this is not a complete reference to the scope of this great treatment program.

Immune System and Vital Power

The Naturopathy believe that human immune system is not just a guard or defender rather it is a master healer and ever builder of body. Naturopathy and Homeopathy are allowing the body and its Vital power to do its own healing by boosting its power using various natural sources around us like water, sun and air. Naturopathy diet allows the body to detoxify and cleanse the system to function efficiently. Yoga, simple exercise and a happy environment are some essential part of this treatment along with prescribed vegetarian diets. According to Dr. Paulose Mar Greegorious in his book "Healing a Holistic Approach" says that our Vital power is the most technically advance system in this universe than any other medical therapy instrument.

Scientists have learned much about the immune system, they continue to study how the body launches attacks that destroy invading microbes, infected cells, and tumors while ignoring healthy tissues. New technologies for identifying individual immune cells are now letting scientists quickly determine which targets are triggering an immune response. Improvements in microscopy are permitting the first-ever observations of B cells, T cells, and other cells as they interact within lymph nodes and other body tissues.

In addition, scientists are rapidly unraveling the genetic blueprints that direct the human immune response as well as those that dictate the biology of bacteria, viruses, and parasites. The combination of new technology and expanded genetic information will no doubt teach us even more about how the body protects itself from disease.

[http://www.imgt.org/IMGTeducation/Tutorials/ImmuneSystem/UK/the_immune_system.pdf]

Some Basic things to Remember and follow for a healthy life recommends by Naturopathy Gurus

- *If you're not hungry do not eat*
- *if you are sick do not eat or reduce eating substantially*
- *Bloating is one of the main cause of many diseases so eat food with lots of fiber; vegetables, fruits and also drink water accordingly*
- *Yoga, exercise, walking, dancing, sports, gardening are some of the main health building process you have to follow to keep fit*
- *Sleep two hours before 12 in midnight, it will help to rebuild the body*
- *Eat slowly and chew the food properly*
- *Every meal should be taken when you are really hungry, if you are not hungry do not eat.*
- *Do not drink water while eating but soup or vegetable juice can be taken with food*

- *Do not eat at night between 10PM and 6AM in the morning.*
- *Do not eat while watching TV or working, should give good attention and respect to food. Eating is an important process to sustains a healthy life.*
- *Take half an hour rest after each meal, if you work without a proper rest and plan it will eventually destroy your organs*
- *Do not sleep immediate after the night meal, ideal sleeping time is minimum two hours after the night meal.*

[A life without disease, Dr. Jacob Vadakkanchery, Page 174]

Food and Health

The eminent teacher of Yoga Govindan Nair says in his book Yoga Padavlai that food got has a greater part to keep us healthy in our life. Food can help us mean time it can trouble us if we use it wrongly. What we are eating how many times we are eating how much quantity we are consuming all these are important factors to keep us healthy. Also do not drink water with food or immediately after the food, the ideal time to consume water is one hour before or after the food. Also it is important to keep in mind that do not eat till you feel full, keep 25% of stomach capacity empty it can be filled with vegetable juice or soup.

[Sri. Yogacharya Govindan Nair, Yoga Padavali]

Quotes

A wise man should consider that health is the greatest of human blessings, and learn how by his own thought to derive benefit from his illnesses. Hippocrates

http://www.brainyquote.com/quotes/quotes/h/hippocrate398538.html

If you have money you can hire someone to drive your car but you cannot hire someone to take your illness that is killing, you.

The last words of Steve Jobs

Naturopathy Study centers in India

If someone want to take this as a career there are study centers in India as follows.

Institutes

There are 10 degree colleges in India that offer the BNYS program, which is of four and half year's duration with a one-year internship.

A look at some colleges and institutes in India that offer naturopathy related courses:

Central Council for Research in Yoga and Naturopathy
(Department of Ayurveda, Yoga & Naturopathy, Unani, Siddha and Homoeopathy)
61-65, Institutional Area, Janakpuri, Phankha Road
New Delhi-110058
Ph.: 91-11-28520430, 91-11-28520431, 91-11-28520432,
Fax: 91-11-28520435
E-mail:ccryn@nda.vsnl.net.in
Website: www.ccryn.org

http://www.indiaeducation.net/careercenter/medical/naturo
pathy/

Bibliography

Books quoted are mentioned at the main frames of this work and also mentioning below for the benefit for someone interested to read more on this great way of life Naturopathy.

1. Sri. R R Varma, Sukam Sathyam, Rogam Madhya

2. Sri. R R Varma, Prekrithi Geevana Chinthakal

3. Sri. N Venkitakrishan Potty, Roogangalilude Poorna Aarogathilekku

4. Dr. Jacob Vadakkanchery, Roogam Illatha Geevitham

5. Dr. Paulos Mar Gregorios, Healing a Holistic Approch

6. Sri. Yogacharya Govinden Nair, Yoga Padavai.